Don't
Be a Dumbell

PHILIPPE DAVIS

ABOUT ME

As a personal trainer with over 10 years experience in the industry and 24 years training under my belt, I have worn many different caps in my lifetime, from working with mental health to occupational therapy to personal training as well as a short stint in natural competitive bodybuilding. It was during a challenge for myself when I came up with the idea to write this book so as to help as many people struggling with understanding true fitness and health on a whole.

I will also add that I do not hold a medical degree and cannot be considered a doctor of any kind. My real passion lies in seeing people improve and live the life they deserve.

WHAT IS THIS BOOK ABOUT?

This book reflects my own lived experience, and the topics of conversations are based from a non-judgmental perspective. There are studies that still remain inconclusive, with subjects such as poor diet being a direct correlation to the cause of endometriosis. Needless to say that a healthy, balanced diet would always be advised considering any underlying conditions.

This book is a guide to healthy eating, understanding carbohydrates, self-improvement, building confidence and

getting over our insecurities. My intention is not to single out anyone who may have underlying conditions, as mentioned in the book. Instead I aim to highlight, risk factors that can be exacerbated if underlying conditions are not taken into serious consideration

In this book I often talk about women and men, female and male physiology. When I do so, I refer to people's sex assigned at birth, not their gender.

Content page

ABOUT ME ii

WHAT IS THIS BOOK ABOUT? iii

Content page iv

DON'T BE FU#k!NG LAZY! 1

CHANGING OLD HABITS A WEEK AT A TIME 4

CONFIDENCE VS. INSECURITY 13

THE LOVE AND HATE FOR FOOD 18

WHY DO I EAT LIKE THIS? 23

UNDERSTANDING FOOD 27

LET'S TALK ABOUT THE SECRET SEASONING 32

UNDERSTANDING SUGAR 43

KING OF THE LIFTS 63

LET'S TALK SUPPLEMENTS... 66

Reference Page 72

DON'T BE FU#k!NG LAZY!

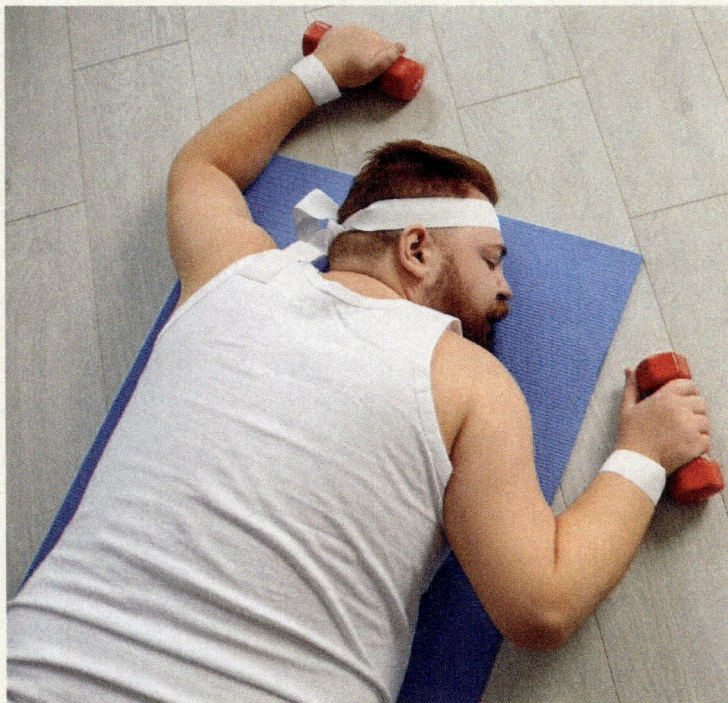

Okay, so this may not be for some of you, but before you close the eBook or shut your brain off, hear me out. When it comes to improving your fitness, or reaching your goals, tell me something: Have you done enough? Honestly? Before you answer: "Yes, I go to the gym twice a week, I have a Personal Trainer, I eat healthy, but I just can't seem to change!

"Consider a few things. Whenever you train, have you set

out your clear objectives for the day? If what you did last week was the same routine as this week, have you made adjustments? How do you know you have improved? Have you and your personal trainer sat down and decided on clear goals for the day?...Are you both keeping each other accountable in tracking your progress?...When it comes to meeting your goals? Your personal trainer only spends so many hours with you per week, so it is very easy for them to not pay serious attention to your progress. You will definitely need to ask for feedback on how well they feel you are improving. I'd say train with you a minimum of 1 and a maximum of 10 hours, which leaves you with 167 or 157 hours per week with full autonomy for yourself. There is only so much your personal trainer can do, and at some point you will need to take full responsibility for your own development.

For example, if you only use a personal trainer twice a week, and don't come to the gym on any other day, then... I'm sorry to tell you this, you are being Lazy! You may say: "I'm just too busy with work/or children/ dinner/ husband/wife/ significant other." or, "I'm so tired when I get home, I just want to unwind or watch TV for an hour or two from my stressful day." Listen, you're making excuses and again you're being lazy!

If you are at work from 9 AM and you finish at around 5 PM. Instead of going home, getting your gym kit, then heading to the gym, Why not take your kit with you to work? Or join the gym near your work place. Train during your lunch break, it doesn't even have to be a super intense workout. Go put on your walking trainers and go out for 40 minutes. Do some straight walking, without a break or change of pace for 40 minutes, then when you come back, grab something to eat and chill for 20 minutes. You see, if you want something bad enough, you'll prepare for it.

I always use the analogy that if I was going on a holiday and had to pay X amount for my trip, plus holiday spending money. I must budget and save until the day of my holiday. When everything is paid for, then I will know that on the day I am ready to fly out, all the hard work is fully complete, all that is left is to enjoy the holiday. This is how we should look at our fitness goals, set the goal, make the sacrifices and bank the benefits.

When you get home, do your chores and if you have children, cater to them first. Then once you have time, grab that skipping rope and skip for 40 minutes, or download a YouTube video and do a full body workout for 40 minutes. Walk up and down some flights of steps. Do something to build up a good sweat within 40 minutes and burn some calories beyond what you'd normally do in your day to day life. Remove those excuses and remember the saying,

"Whether you think you can, or can't... you're right"

▶ Bo Talley Williams (77 years old) Comp…

CHANGING OLD HABITS A WEEK AT A TIME

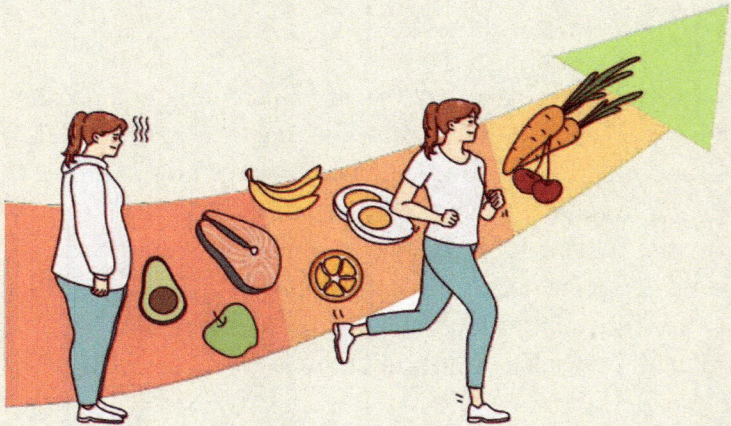

If you're someone who hasn't been to the gym in a long time, or never been to the gym at all. You may have fallen into one of these categories: You may have fallen into a comfort zone of doing the same habits every day. You could be relatively fit, or not. If you are easily motivated, but a lot of time, your consistency may have fallen off.

You may be in the habit of waking up for work at 6/7AM in the morning for work or maybe you don't even need to go work but you just feel like getting up whenever you feel like it.

Well I offer you a fun little challenge for yourself: Set your alarm 15 minutes earlier than you normally would, and within that 15 minutes do something, not necessarily training related but just something in preparation to make your day go easier. Make lunch, answer a quick email, iron the kids uniform, meditate. Do something productive for that extra 15 minutes you've woken up with.

Do this for 1 week, then the next week, do something different say 10 Squats every morning as you get up then go do your new routine, just still keeping within your 15 minutes. Then the week after that do 20 Squats every day, it doesn't even have to be Squats, it could be star jumps. By slowly changing your pattern and making your mind more productive, that extra 15 minutes will add up to 3 hours 40 minutes in a month. You will notice the changes over time and from there take your time to expand on your new routine. (It takes the human brain between 18 days to 9 weeks and 2.5 months for anything to become a natural habit) After this point it almost becomes second nature.

https://youtube.com/shorts/2FlUQKAHgPQ?feature=share

NO MAN IS AN ISLAND

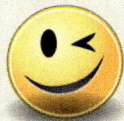

I am amazing, there's no denying this fact; I wake up 4:30AM, go do my cardio after making my breakfast, train my clients between 6 and 10 A.M, train myself for an hour, then go on to train some more clients throughout the day and at the end of the day go home to

5

play with my beautiful daughter and amazing family...

Yeah, that's complete bullsh!t.

The truth is, I would not be able to complete half of my daily activities without support from my wife. She would cook some of my meals, she'd give me encouraging words to remind me not to give up on a project. Even with the fact that she spends 80 percent of her time taking care of our daughter and giving me the freedom to operate, is the best kind of support I could ever ask for. I also need accountability, that my children keep me held to. Yes, both my children keep me accountable. My daughter will remark "daddy your tummy is getting bigger" if she feels that I am getting a little out of shape. This always helps to keep an eye on those cheat meals (there's nothing like a child's brutal honesty to keep you in check).

My son has asked me one of the most important questions that I have ever been asked in recent years. Not that I haven't been asked this before, but when your child makes a statement or asks you a question, any person worth their salt will want to answer as honestly and earnestly as possible.

He asked me "Dad, how much longer will you be doing the career that you are doing?"

Which gave me a good pause, because in all honesty I did not give it any serious thought until he asked, but his question prompted me to look for new avenues and life goals to work toward. It caused me to look inward and take stock, as I knew he was asking from a place of true curiosity and concern for my wellbeing.

You see, if you have a good support network around you, it'll make your goals ten times easier and achievable. When the people around you are able to understand your goal, even if they don't share them, their support can help you complete yours. Your friends can also help along the way, as well as people who doubt that you can progress. Yes, those who'd doubt you, can also be a good driving factor, especially if you don't really like that person's opinion of you. Use that negative feedback to prove them wrong.

So you too can become amazing like me.

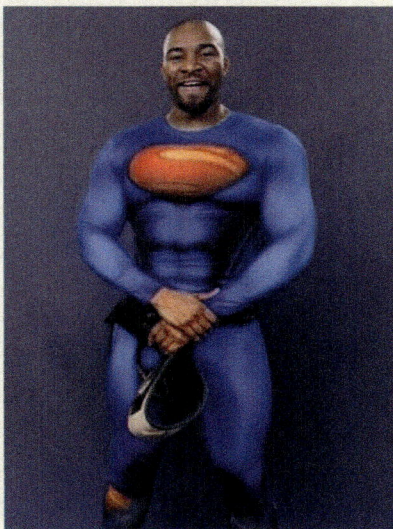

So you've decided to come back to the gym. You think to yourself: "Bloody Hell, this is all a bit too much, too new, too intimidating for me. I want to lose a bit of weight, but what can I do? The best thing you can do, when starting back at the gym, is find a like-minded friend, to become a gym buddy.

Don't go for that buff, super fit friend to motivate you!

This could be a bad idea for several reasons:

1. You don't want to intimidate yourself further. If your friend's fitness level is above your own, you may end up feeling like you're being dragged along, while trying to train with them. Now, while this can and will boost their confidence, it'll do very little for your self esteem.

While training with a strong friend, they may be a bit more bossy, less friendly, less motivational and more like a bootleg Personal Trainer. If the both of you don't know much about training, but your partner may know a little bit more than you, you may even end up listening to incorrect, bad advice. Though it may well work for them, it could lead to impingement, and injuries for you.

2. Your friend may not understand that you're not on their level yet. You may need to have someone that you can have a connection with. I don't mean a romantic or even necessarily a friendship, but a connection where you both have the same goals in mind, you both know that you need to change something, you both understand the intimidation of the gym so therefore will be able to support each other.

But let's be real and don't get confused. When you go to

the gym with someone as a training partner, your goals may be similar, or the motivation may be there for both of you, but ultimately you are there for yourself! Don't depend on that person to always have the same reason for training in mind, because everyone has issues that they need to work through. Albeit life, work stress, confidence, (jealousy, oh yes!) If you respond well while working out, but your new gym friend doesn't see changes in their physique for some reason, that green eyed monster can creep in. Negative comments here and there, may be dropped in conversation, they may start training less and less.

Don't be fooled, even your super fit friend might get jealous. When these types of differences start to happen, like in any relationship, it's time to address/change or separate. I liken this scenario to a car journey. We get into a car going from point A to point Z, but if at some point your companion wants to keep stopping at D, E & F, then that journey is not for you. It will slow your progress, or side track you. Get out, and get back on track! You don't have to go to the gym with a friend, you can make new ones at the gym. Most gyms will have some type of classes going on.

Go check some classes out, sit and watch from the back of a class. Whilst doing your workout, you'll be able to see who the super fit people are, the people who struggle, the people who are confident.

Look for a common interest among people, there may be something that you notice about the instructor, or the music that's being played. Pay attention to little conversations in the changing rooms afterwards, about the class. Try to pick up a general vibe of the people around you. Now you definitely don't have to join in conversations straight away. In fact, you may come across a bit too strong, if you try to jump in on someone's conversation, someone you've just seen for the first time.

It takes 5 times of seeing someone on 5 separate occasions before we can build familiarity. It is from this point, that we can potentially start a natural organic conversion or introduction without seeming pushy, nosey, odd or genuinely misunderstood.

Anything before the point of introduction should really be "Hi", glance and smile. You can workout if a person is friendly, or does not wish to interact at all, using this strategy. If someone chooses not to engage at all, try to remember that they may be as nervous as you, or may even harbour insecurities of their own. Generally most people can be stuck in their own bubble of emotions, and will find a group of like-minded people they can feel safe and comfortable around.

If classes are not your thing, then you can do what I call "the cardio watcher game", but try not to get stuck in this mode, as it's a very easy default mode to get stuck in. Cardio Watcher Game: You come into the gym, jump on a piece of cardio equipment potentially for 5-20 minutes. During this time, you watch the culture of the gym.

Take note of the people to avoid, the people who are friendly, loud and confident, and the people there just like you. Take note of other people who may be nervous, who don't necessarily know what they are doing, so they

10

will have jumped on a piece of cardio equipment as well. They may be wearing headphones to overcome interaction. Remember the 5 times rule is also important while playing the cardio game with all these types of people. Talking is only 1 form of communication, and not necessarily the first form of communication.

Remember that the cardio game has to end at some point and avoid doing your cardio longer than 20 minutes at a time. This is just a warm up, there is no need to do crazy sprints or a vigorous workout, whereby you can't even talk. If someone asks you a question. You want to be able to have a conversation while doing the cardio game. This is a Potential tactic used to meet like minded people, or someone who you can train with.

If The Cardio Watcher Game is not your thing, and you don't like classes, you can always find a Personal Trainer. This will give you more accountability as well as confidence, since you get your guidance from a professional.

But remember, that your personal trainer is only part of your journey to achieve your overall goal at the gym. Whilst there are many other options and ways of training, the reason I have mentioned the above in this way is to keep your interaction and relationship with the gym as organic as possible. while helping to build your confidence, without making obvious that you are new to, or just starting back up at the gym.

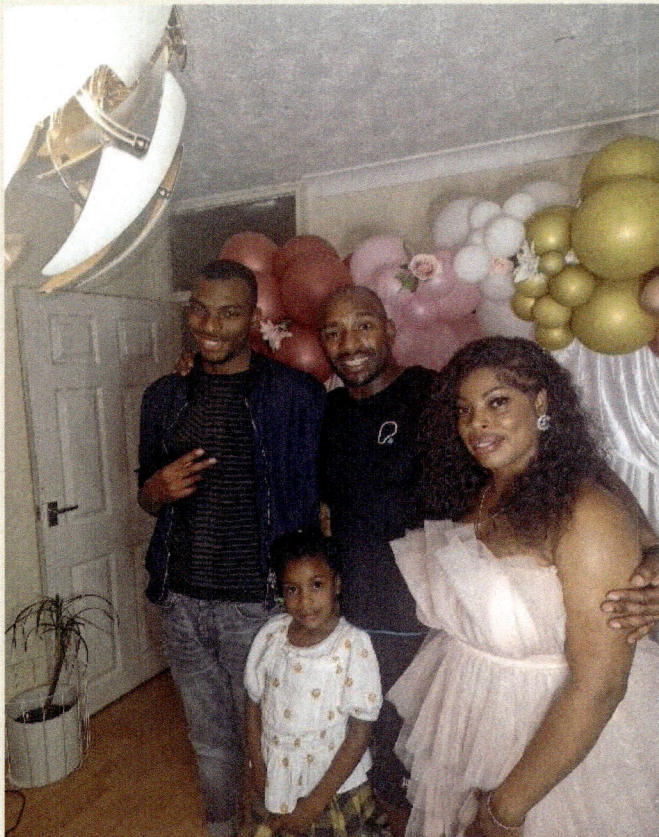

CONFIDENCE VS. INSECURITY

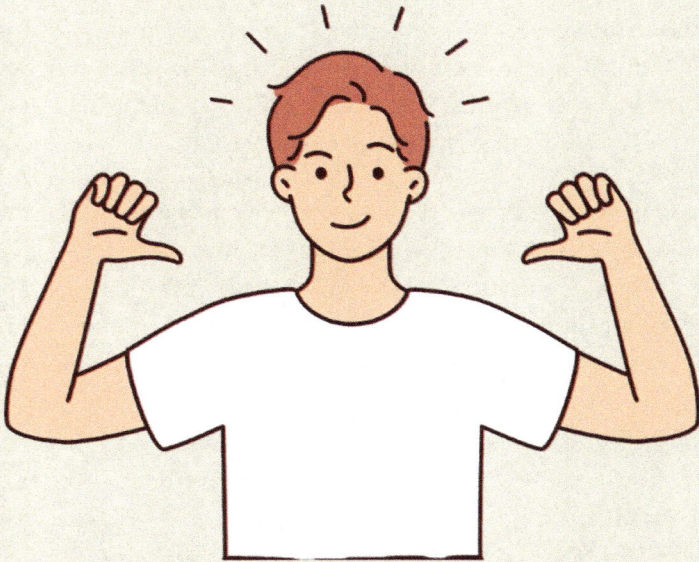

Let me tell you a story. As the last child to 4 sisters and 1 brother, I grew up in a very active household. My mum is very knowledgeable and a strong character. She is confident as well as charismatic and a role model to a lot of women in the early 80s. Mum had friends from all over the world. People would come from all over to get advice on work, relationships and home life. What ways were best to deal with unfair employment & management.

Whether you were gay, straight, young or old, if you had just come into the country or had been a citizen all your life; Mum knew it all and had answers for everyone. I thought my mum was the smartest lady I had ever seen.

It really hurt me on the day I heard her comparing me with my nephew. I was playing in the hallway downstairs, and I could hear my sister and mum speaking about my nephew, who was 3 years younger than me. She was saying that I wasn't as smart as him, nor did I show as much potential. This didn't really bother me much, as I was just a 7 year old And being smart wasn't a priority to me in those days.

It was only the day when I was on a visit around my grandmother's house, with a few of my cousins and 1 of my nephews that I learned a valuable lesson. My grandmother took her bible out and called me over. She opened this huge book and said "Read this passage, Pickny!" I took one look at all these words, which at the time didn't mean anything to me and said "I can't read, Granny". Her eyes widened and her jaw dropped, time seemed to stand still. At this point all my siblings who were in the room at the time, turned and started laughing.

They took out magazine's and were pointing to words saying "read this!"And how do you spell "THE?, how do you spell CAT?, " Every time I said "I don't know", they'd roll over doubled in laughter.

This was confirmation that my mother was right and that I was stupid. (Oh, it was as brutal and embarrassing as only a 7-year-old could experience, at that point in time). This still never bothered me much, as I knew my Mum

loved me very much. She'd always call me over to sit on

her bed with her at random times, give me the biggest hugs, pinch the end of my nose and say "You're so handsome with your big brown eyes."

This made me feel so special. It was only when my sister (the brain-box of the family) came back from America, and found out that I couldn't read, that I realised the importance, and the big differences between my nephew and myself. But my sister would soon close the gap, by teaching me how to read. She would make these word searches, and created spelling games. We would play hangman, and do crossword puzzles. My middle sister Angela, who was my most influential sister, would ask me "What do you want to be, when you're old Phil?" Me being a 7 year old, who really hadn't thought past the end of the day would reply "I don't know" and shrug. My sister would then continue and say "You can be anything that you want to, you know. A pilot, a fireman. Why don't you become a policeman? I can see you doing that."

What I didn't know then, but learned later on, is that my 2 sisters and my mum are my role models. They formed my insecurities, as well as my confidence. I also learned that my Mum didn't actually know it all. Nor was she right about everything... No matter how many qualifications I acquire, or how much praise I get about my knowledge in particular subjects, my insecurities will, to this day, easily take me back to those days of being teased. My mum's conversation will be ringing in my ears, I will instantly feel dumb again, thinking about every time I failed an exam, or got an answer wrong.

To overcome these emotions, as an adult I had to take

ownership, and realise that my insecurities were something only I could see and know about. You see, that's the thing about our insecurities, only you know what they are. Not one other person will be able to tell, unless you show them what you are insecure about, it's not through admitting that we have issues, but through our reactive behaviour in situations that make us feel uncomfortable. For me, if someone pointed out a spelling mistake I made, I'd start to feel my palms go clammy. I'd also start making excuses, as to why the mistake was made, or I'd take offence to questions of dyslexia. I'd over elaborate, when asked any question. I would study twice as hard on subjects I enjoyed, just to prove to myself that I was smart. I realised that nobody actually cared about my insecurities as much as I did, because they were too busy dealing with their own.

You can only face your insecurities by owning them, and the more you try to hide or avoid them, the more they may grow. It is only when you can say f*ck it, I'm the only one who can see you, so therefore I own you. That's when you can actually start to be free, and move on with your life.

One of the ways I'd prove to myself that I had potential for academics, I went back to school. I retook my GCSEs. This was while my son was in secondary school. He gave me the drive to do more and keep on going, because even though I could help him with his homework, I couldn't help but feel like a fraud without those qualifications. So I went back and quietly did my retakes. While at night school, I also got tested too, and it turned out that I didn't have dyslexia. I would have never found this out unless I faced my insecurities. You see, for me it was the embarrassment of not completing my G.C.S.Es while my son was about to achieve his. To this day it remains such a huge lesson, as to why we must face our insecurities.

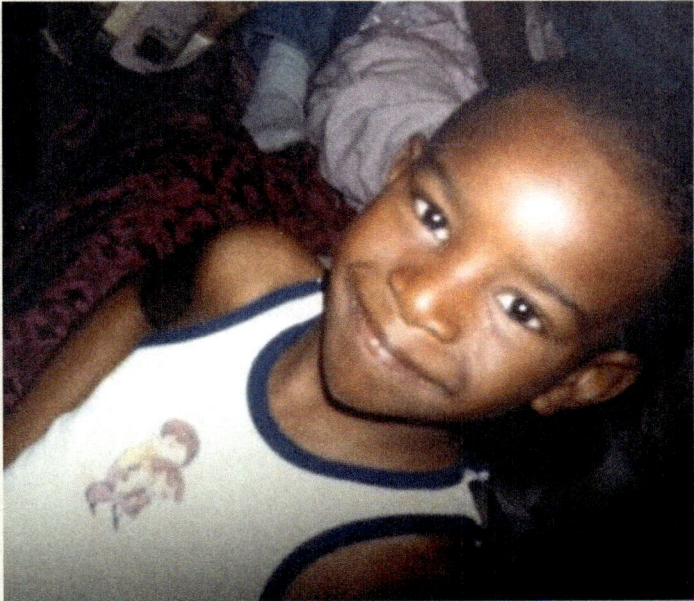

THE LOVE AND HATE FOR FOOD

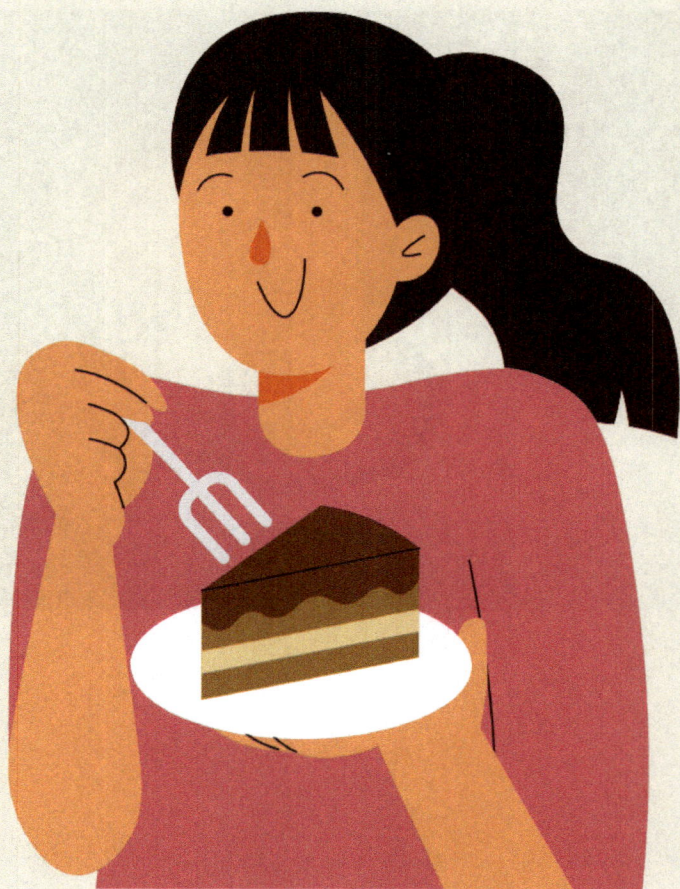

When I was a child of about 6 years old in the 80s, my Dad and I used to take trips through Peckham every Saturday. We'd stop at the local bakery, where my dad would say to me:"Pick out what cake you want" I'd usually pick out the cupcake with a picture on it, or the iced finger (sometimes even 2). Dad would always laugh loudly and say "You dun dem already!" Surprised at the speed I had eaten them.

This was our "Thing". We'd then go on to McDonald's, where Dad would buy me a root beer, chocolate ring doughnut, chips and a cheeseburger. Till this day I'd always get a cupcake with the picture on it or an iced finger & the staff in Gregs would laugh at the sight of a 40-something-year-old man eating a child's cupcake.

Until recently I had been putting on weight due to me buying lots of takeaway food, more specifically Nigerian foods like pounded yam and stew. My wife would cook these wonderful Caribbean meals for dinner, but I'd always come home with Nigerian takeaway. She would be confused and sometimes upset. she'd ponder as to why I came home, laid out the food on the floor, and went through the ritual of washing my hands before eating my food without cutlery, just as I did when I was a child. I had been doing this so often that my daughter would come to join me. In fact you can say that it has become our little tradition and our "Thing". My wife never understood why and neither did I until recently.

You see, when I was a child, my sister Angela, had loads of Nigerian friends & was a big influence on me. Angie would cook loads of pounded yam and stew meals. She had us all sit in a circle on the floor, to share two big bowls of food after we'd washed our hands to eat in the traditional Nigerian way. Unfortunately my sister died 2 years ago, and it only occurred to me that I'd eat these meals whenever I was stressed, upset or missing her.

Every mouthful of pounded yam and stew would take me back to those days and I'd sit and smile almost as though I was a child again, sitting on the floor with the family. If you're anything like me, you may have formed some really good memories of food. Some foods will remind us of where we ate it the first time, the good or bad experiences we shared with friends or family.

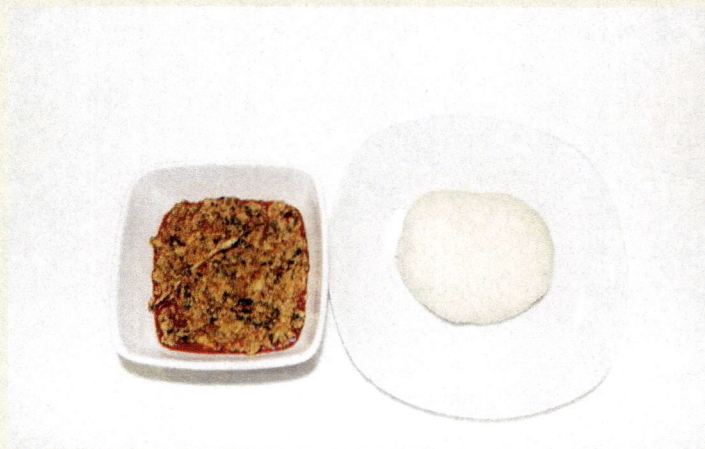

Food can trigger memories of joy, sadness, comfort, just by the smells. We may remember our first time eating with a friend or something bad that was said to us while eating a particular meal.

Have you ever gotten drunk on a particular drink that made you violently ill... what was your reaction every time after seeing or smelling that drink?

Our memories of foods, smells and textures, can even

trigger physical responses without even eating, and will definitely influence our approach to food. Just like alcohol if you had a bad experience. This same trigger also can happen.

Let's say a bad egg, that gave you food poisoning, or your mum forced you to eat sprouts when you were a child. You may need to reintroduce these foods back into your diet slowly, using our senses TASTE, TOUCH, SMELL, SIGHT.

We can even consider the sound of a food E.G. the bubbling of soup or frying of bacon. Try to take time using each of your senses to get acquainted and reintroduce the food that you have issues with back into your diet.

If you hold insecurities about yourself, food can be a much needed comfort blanket when you're stressed. If you start eating as though you need to fill a hole inside, it is at this point that you will need to address the issues as to why you feel the need to comfort eat. This requires a more in depth solution other than just exercise. Seeking counselling or Cognitive Behavioural Therapy (CBT) may be useful tools alongside diet and food education.

Working out can be considered as a form of therapy that will help reduce stress levels. A 20-minute walk, or going for a run, can greatly reduce cortisol, the stress hormone.

Ultimately if you find yourself overeating or not eating enough, because of stress, then it would be a good time to remove yourself from those difficult situations. Then you can regroup your emotions and lower your anxiety for self-preservation. For example, you work for a hard-to-please senior member of management, who demands more than what is needed to complete work deadlines. They never seem pleased or praise you on any work you have completed. Either they blame you for taking too long to complete a project, or they overload you with additional tasks with no consideration. You find that when you need to go to work, you feel a deep anxiety. Once your workday has ended, you feel drained as you lament on comments your boss has made about your work throughout the day. You find that the only thing that can pick your mood up would be to start eating loads of bread and doughnuts, until your stomach is tight and to the point that you feel like vomiting.

You notice that you only go through this pattern of behaviour after working directly under this particular boss.

It is at this point that you may need to request some time off from work to assess your life options. Once you have removed yourself from the trigger of your problems, you can now strategize, about what would be the logical way to deal with the issues you are having.

Many of us come to an important crossroads in our lives, where we may have to make the choice of what we regard more as a priority, our mental health, or our lifestyle.

WHY DO I EAT LIKE THIS?

foodies

Pro Tip: NEVER! shop for food when you are hungry, you will always buy what you crave at the time and not what you actually need.

We always make bad decisions while shopping while hungry. Make a list before you set out and have a budget in mind. Also eat before you enter wherever you're going to buy your food. gas stove. And just in case there weren't enough vegetables, there would be coleslaw, and a tub of homemade salad all from scratch.

Okay, so I've mentioned a few times that I'm from a

Caribbean background and grew up in the 80s. It is traditional in a West Indian household to have Sunday be a big thing. My mum being a catering chef, this was definitely no exception. Every Sunday I'd wake up to the smell of rice and peas being cooked on the pressure cooker, the mix of coconut cream in the rice would hit you like no other.

Mum would be down in the kitchen, cooking up a storm. With fried chicken, roast lamb, jerk pork, roast potatoes, plantain, a melody of asparagus, courgettes, carrot,

cabbage in the wok and the gravy pot bubbling on the open Mum would be in there for what seemed like ages from the morning til around 12 midday. (Not joking, this was every Sunday dinner in our household). We were a household of 6 at the time, but we'd get a visit from my uncle Ben and aunt Cynthia, who'd come around most Sundays. Even my uncle Junior who would take enough food to last him a week. When it came to dinner time mum would pile my plate high with this mountain of rice, despite me saying "Only one spoon please mum." Then would come the chicken, lamb, pork, potatoes and veg. As a 7-year-old this was so overwhelming, I'd say "I can't eat all of this mum! " to which she'd replied "Eat what you can and throw the rest away". When it came to my dad's portion, he would eat what could only be described as a tray of food, with what looked like a small pot spoon.

He would sit on his bed with his pint glass full of coke mixed with milk and ice, shovelling these heaps of hot food in his mouth and sweating from the hot pepper sauce. Needless to say, dinner was never a problem for dad to eat. When it came to mum's diet, her average meal would be a plate full of all these vegetables, and a separate bowl full of rice, with one of every kind of meat she had cooked that day. I'd watch mum struggling to eat her own food. She would eat as much as she could, put the tray down at her bedside and continue eating later in the day, while wrapping the food up until the meal was finished.

The funny thing is, she'd also eat other things during the day, but would never throw the food away. It wasn't until I became older and could give it some thought into mum's strange eating habits, why didn't she just throw the food away? I mean that's what she told me and my siblings to do, and believe me we did just that. To this day, we are the only family in our area who have 4 black wheelie bins and 2 recycling bins.

You see, where my mum came from in Jamaica, food may have been scarce. So when you get the opportunity to cook and eat, you'd eat till your belly is full, as it may be your only meal for the day. My mum learned the habit as a child that food was not to be wasted. Being a protector/matriarch of the family, subconsciously she only wanted to provide for her family and not let us go through what she may have experienced as a child.

She also didn't realise that giving me these heaps of food had the opposite effect that it had on her. Fortunately, she was able to give me some balance by allowing me to eat as much as I could handle and throw the rest away. If you were like me, and your parents worked hard to provide food for dinner, you may have been given these unhealthy subliminal phrases to consider as well. "Eat your food, there are children starving in Africa".

Back then you'd be eating dinner, while watching the Red Cross advert with these unfortunate children with swollen bellies, and force yourself to eat another spoonful of rice thinking, I'll eat for the both of us mate.

Your parents may have been quite the opposite to mine and made you feel bad for being hungry or wanting more food. With phrases like who ate all the pies while poking your tummy. I can only imagine if you were an impressionable child/teenager growing up going through puberty and your body going through these hormonal changes, the last thing you want to hear is anything to do with your weight or how much that you should be eating. Especially if you get a spike in ghrelin (the hunger hormone) telling you "if you don't eat now

I'm going to pinch the Hell out of you, until you go insane". When it came to food, in most Caribbean and African households the issue was never what we ate, but that the portions were always too much.

It's okay to be hungry and leave a little space in your tummy. In fact, you may even enjoy your food more.

UNDERSTANDING FOOD

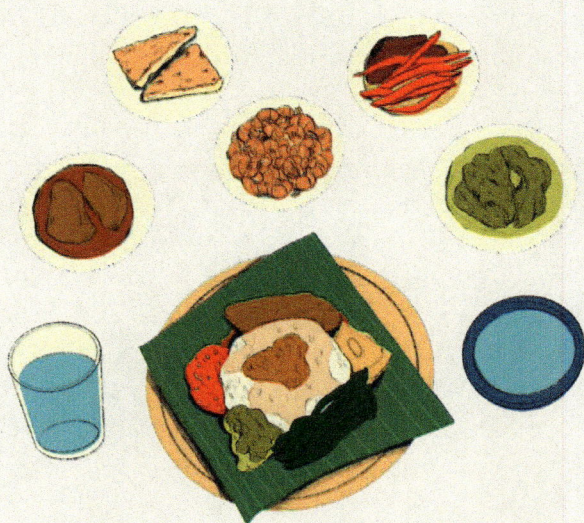

So you're trying to lose inches and think "I know what I'll do, I'll go on a diet!" So you do so. Diet for 6, 7, X amount of weeks, lose some inches or pounds, only to put twice as much back on once you have achieved your goal. Here are the problems with this: You have to understand that your diet is for life, and not just for X amount of time which you choose to lose weight. You can starve your body of calories only for so long, before your (BMR) basal metabolic rate is affected.

This is the minimum amount of calories your body needs to operate at rest during your sleep. If you try to drop your body below these calories your body will automatically go into starvation mode, and after a while hold on to every calorie you eat. In-turn,you will be resetting your BMR to a new point. In the meantime you'll feel like crap as well lose muscle volume. At this point the whole ordeal of eating can become an unenjoyable experience. So what do I do then... get a diet plan? Eat no carbs after 7PM? Cut carbs completely? Do intermittent fasting? As I've said before, your diet is for life. unless you plan to do intermittent fasting for the rest of your life, then that is not the answer.

Now using fasting in terms of cardiovascular exercise, or resistance training... This is completely different. **(Pro tip:** When you train/do your cardio on an empty stomach you will burn fat, whereas when you train/do your cardiovascular exercise on a full stomach you'll burn calories.)** Eating no carbohydrates after 7PM only makes sense, only if you're not active at all after 7PM. Plus carbohydrates are in everything so trying to eat no carbohydrates is impossible. The most logical answer is to learn how carbohydrates work. Understanding what complex carbohydrates are vs simple carbohydrates.

The easiest way to understand how this works is, any food that is hard to eat (chew) unprocessed (natural state) will be classed as complex carbohydrates. Potatoes, yam, wholegrain or brown rice, sweet potatoes, are all examples of the perfect complex carbs. They will take longer in the body to digest, so in turn the body will use energy breaking them down in the stomach to extract the sugar content for energy and convert to glucose.

More simple carbohydrates are all your foods that can easily be eaten and digested really quickly, and convert to glucose much quicker. They are always processed and high in sugar. The body does not need to do much work at all converting these foods into energy. Therefore they will boost sugar/glucose levels fast and they will metabolise to fat much easier. White rice (husk removed), mashed potatoes (skin removed), any kind of pasta, any kind of bread. All these types of carbs are considered as starchy carbohydrates. All kinds of cereal! Granola especially will fall into the category of simple starchy carbohydrates!

Once you can understand what is complex and what is simple, you can plan your workout/working day more effectively. Remember you still can enjoy both, just think of it as using the right type of fuel, to do the right types of jobs at the right points of the day. If you're going to have a really busy day that tapers down leading into the night, it makes sense to eat your simple carbs as you'll need that energy.

But when it comes to the end of that busy day you'll want your carbohydrates to be as low or little as possible. All vegetables would be excellent at completing this within a meal, especially cruciferous vegetables. Broccoli, asparagus, cabbage, courgettes, spinach, brussel sprouts are some examples of the most common and best vegetables, they are very low in carbohydrates and also rich in vitamins, minerals, and antioxidants. All are considered fibrous carbohydrates.

Here are some key tips to cut ghrelin(the hunger

hormone):<u>ghrelin</u>

- Increase your protein

- Increase you good fats

- Set up a regular eating pattern, try not eating until you are bursting full, and always leave space for more

- Drink plenty of water so you know the hunger that you are feeling is actually hunger and not dehydration

Got a sweet tooth. Here are some of my favourite snacks to provide energy, cut ghrelin and promote fat loss.

1. **Watermelon**: Sweet and very low in calories at 30 calories per 100 grams. The fibre produced and the minerals will help to decrease blood pressure. There are also antioxidants that will reduce inflammation and infection.

2. **Berries**: Blueberries, raspberries, black berries. While all are low in carbohydrate and high in fibre, as well as being very sweet, these fruits are rich in antioxidants, and extremely versatile.

3. **Dark chocolate**: Anything above 80% coco for me is a win. Rich in magnesium, high in good fats, and a good source of energy that will cut ghrelin. This snack is one of my favourite go-tos in times of need to cut hunger.

4. **Almond butter or peanut butter**: Most nuts are

a good snack. However these two come with so much more benefits, with almond butter being rich in magnesium, protein, vitamin E and lowering blood sugar, this snack is perfect for people with diabetes. Plus if you are worried about the calories, powdered peanut butter carries half the calories of normal peanut butter.

(when buying any of these two butters make sure that you see the oils floating on the top and avoid the hydrogenated versions)

Snack hacks:

Dark chocolate and peanut butter together are such an amazing mix that peanut butter cups should be illegal.

Frozen, blended berries with lemon juice and a teaspoon of honey make the best sorbet, and you can add watermelon to add a sweeter taste.

(Even though these snacks are now home processed they still will hold a nutritional value and still convert to glucose, but can't be considered as simple sugars)

LET'S TALK ABOUT THE SECRET SEASONING

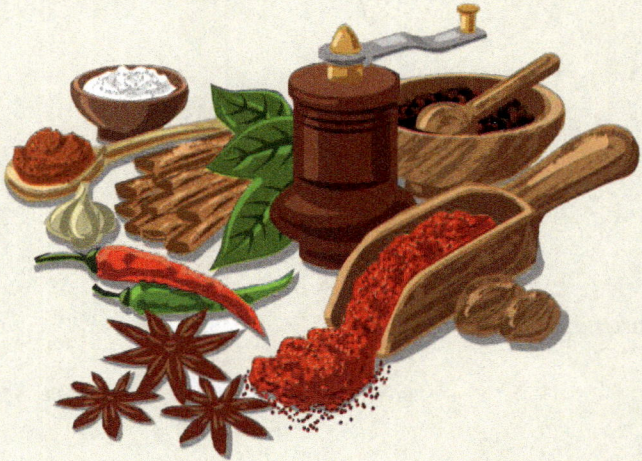

What if I told you that there is a seasoning out there, that is the cocaine of all seasonings. It was created in 1908 by professor Ikedia, and blew up in the late 1970s, just like cocaine. It became extremely popular amongst Chinese takeaways due to its moorish taste.

Nowadays, it's in nearly all the fast foods and snacks that we eat. From biscuits to crisps, noodles and soups. In fact, a lot of Caribbean households would use this seasoning, because of its ability to make your food 10 times more tasty, by stimulating your dopamine receptors (the pleasure hormone.)The name of this seasoning is Monosodium Glutamate, or M.S.G. also known as Seasoning Salt. This seasoning produces a salty/savoury, almost but not quite sweet taste known as Umami. There are three foods that produce the taste of Umami naturally: mushrooms, tomatoes and cheese.

Although this MSG taste is produced naturally in these 3 foods, it can also be found in foods such as: hydrolyzed vegetable protein, autolyzed yeast, hydrolyzed yeast, yeast extract, soy extracts, and protein isolate. All of which will undergo processing to make the food last longer. This process causes food to become carcinogenic, by changing the food's molecules so that the product's ageing process is delayed naturally. So as you can see, here lies the problem. We have this addictive taste, produced by this amazing seasoning. When extracted it is pretty good by itself, but when added to unhealthy foods it will not only make them taste very good, but also make them somewhat addictive. So now that you know the colonel's secret, What will you do about it?...

Seasonings that should be a must in 90% of our foods

1. Garlic with its anti-inflammatory properties. Garlic is also low calorie and in some foods the combination is amazing (garlic mushrooms always has that wow factor for me)

2. Ginger also is an anti inflammatory and tastes so nice in combination with most, if not all of your dark greens and leafy vegetables

Rosemary works wonders with pork, beef, chicken, duck,

lamb and it is antioxidant, and antimicrobial

3. Thyme goes best with carrots, goat cheese, tomatoes, onions and pork

4. Parsley is another antioxidant that works well with all white fish

5. Lemon is good for weight loss, it is antibacterial and it tastes good with all fish, muscles, crab, and in fact with most seafood. It is excellent to clean chicken, fish, lemon, it will kill E.coli, salmonella, listeria (so always clean your chicken and fish with lemon or vinegar, before cooking)

INFLAMMATION IN THE BODY

Okay so, if you're like me, you don't mind eating a sausage , or a chocolate bar once in a while. I'm of the belief that all foods have a purpose, and can be used in some way to benefit your body. However there are some foods that remain carcinogenic to our bodies and will do much more harm than good. These foods will not only cause inflammation in your body but contribute to the destruction of your health. **cereals**

All cereals are nothing but high processed carbohydrates sugar, which are easily digestible and carry no nutritional value other than high fibre. This is the main reason why I say that cereal can not be classed as a Breakfast. It falls into the category of sweet/snack, likened to eating a bag of crisps or cakes. It is not even as good as popcorn when it comes to nutritional value.

Cereal is not breakfast! The importance of breakfast is to Break a Fast, after not eating for X amount of hours through a 24 hour period, this also can help with ketosis if structured right. Some people even believe that fasting the body for as long as 36 hours will create autophagy, a process whereby the cell ageing is slowed right down, creating longevity and slowing ageing. Autophagy is also recommended in combination with veganism, to help treat early cancer diagnosis, as it is said to starve cancerous cells in the body.

Your first meal should be able to sustain at least your morning and help energise your day the following foods I've listed below remain a no-go area for me, as they will be overly processed, over heat- treated, have too many additives, and simply are cancerous to the body. They contribute to conditions such as P.C.O.S. Gynaecomastia, asthma, diabetes, (endometriosis, *the jury is still out as studies are 100% conclusive*) acne, eczema and most inflammation in your body.

In no particular order:

1. Bacon, smoked or any kind out of a packet **processed meats**

2. Doritos crisps

3. Soy milk, tofu: studies have shown that excessive soy can cause erectile dysfunction (however this needs more research as evidence remains inconclusive). Personally I would still avoid soy, as I have seen issues with male clients consuming excessive amounts of soy milk, and shortly after

developing gynecomastia, for it only to be reduced once stopped.

4.   Cereals

5.   Processed cheese, slices, canned, creamed

6.   Coke (diet or coke zero) may as well drink coke and take the sugar risk.

7.   Beer

8.   Biltong, heat treatment of this meat and the process in the cooking and additional additives, make any kind of packet meats like it carcinogenic

9.   Hydrogenated oils (margarine)

10. Sunflower oils

11. Vegetable oils

12. Mint, (studies from 2014 & 2017 show that mint can lower testosterone levels in women suffering with P.C.O.S.) however The jury is still out on whether it will do the same to men.

In small quantities, the above foods are bad at best. They won't kill you after one meal, but they sure as Hell won't help improve your health. The process used to make these foods, as well as the combination of additives in them, will cause them to become very dangerous / carcinogenic to the body. Well, how can I slow, stop, or reverse inflammation in my body? To me water remains king.

If you're not hitting at least 2 litres of pure water per day you're leaving your body with the high probability of being dehydrated. Headaches, dry mouth, lethargy, bad skin, high blood pressure are all results from lack of water in the body. Changing your food cooking oils will also improve your chances of better health and weight loss, coconut oil and olive oil should be the number one choice to bring down Inflammation in the body. Coconut oil contains MCT (Medium Chain Triglyceride), which will aid in lowering your calorie intake, can be used as an immediate source of energy, as they enter your bloodstream straight away and can be converted into ketones in the liver. This also improves the chances of lowering the risk of Alzheimer's and epilepsy.MCT will help fight yeast and bacterial growth, and can help manage blood sugar levels.

Ginger, garlic, red Onion, Red Cabbage, beetroot, Cranberries, and turmeric are all vegetables you need to add to your daily food intake if you want to bring down Inflammation in the body. Either 1, 2 or all of them in combination will lower blood pressure, help brain function, clear skin, clear mucus in the body, fight bacteria or fight infections. ginger and turmeric sardines, coconut, hemp seeds, walnuts, mushrooms, mackerel, salmon, all will help improve vision brain health and give the right omega 3 & 6 to help brain function. Try eating 1, 2 or all of these in combination once a week and experience how your sleep and thought processing improves.

You don't have to follow or subscribe to anything that I'm saying. In fact there may even be counter-arguments, to disprove what I am saying. Anyone can find in some sort of study or literature, to disagree nower-days.

Quite frankly it is your choice. If all the things you are currently doing have not been working 100% then why not, try these changes for 3 months and see, what do you have to lose?

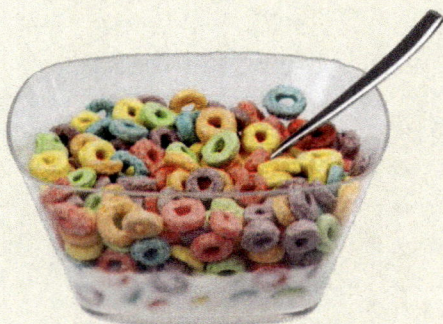

HAVE A DRINK, WHY NOT?

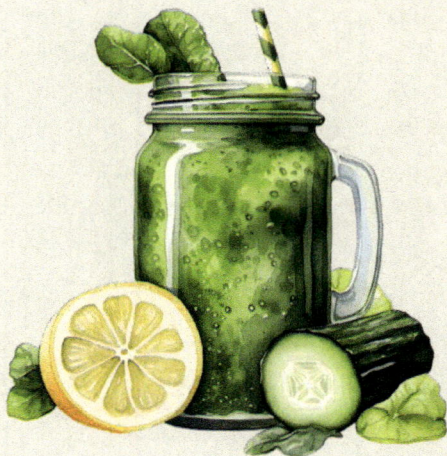

Okay so if you're trying to count calories, but not including what you drink, especially when it comes to alcohol. 2 large glasses of white wine at 250 ml, can set you back 500 calories, 500 ml of vodka calories can total in 1082 and a 500 ml can of cider will be 210 calories. If you take into consideration that all alcohol calories have no nutritional value, besides putting up your blood sugar, it becomes a hard pill to swallow. You may need to ask yourself the question: is drinking this worth increasing my calories? Paired with the fact that, the main chemical in alcohol to get you high is actually toxic.

Ref: DCCEW "Ethanol is harmful by ingestion, inhalation or by skin absorption. Repeated contact can dry the skin resulting in the skin cracking, peeling and itching. Ethanol can depress the central nervous system, the eyes and upper respiratory tract (nose and throat). 30 June 2022"

Ethanol will also shrink your brain, causing black spots in memory. It dries out your liver, has links to Alzheimer's as well as Korsakoff syndrome. This is a shortage of B1 vitamins, causing memory loss from excessive drinking. So maybe the next time you go to have that one social drink with a friend, or on a work dinner, you might just want to do the maths first.

Some drinks we may think are healthy, need to be questioned. Smoothies are an excellent way to get extra nutrients into the body as well as putting on excess calories, if you so wish.

If you struggle with eating, a smoothie can provide a great way to increase calories, however a smoothie is not the entire picture rather a small part of the puzzle. Example of a bad smoothie would be adding bananas and honey, when there is no real need to. Why not just eat a banana, which you will also get fibre from, and burn more calories while masticating, and actually giving your body the chance to work, while digesting your food? Are you adding honey to your smoothie?... Well here is the thing about adding honey... honey in a small amount can be good for your immune system.

5 grams of honey, 1 teaspoon can help improve heart health, lower blood pressure and even aid fat loss. As with anything you consume, if you go over the dose of 1 teaspoon then, you're just eating for flavour. Which leads to the opposite effect, boosting your blood glucose levels therefore doing exactly the same as overeating spoons full of sugar.

If you want to make a tasty drink, that will benefit your body, and contains low calories, opt for juiced watermelon with juiced cucumber and blueberries. This will benefit your skin and improve your libido. Don't go for boxed juices, as the likelihood is they would have preservatives, additives and will be made from a high concentration of the fruit that you believe you are consuming.

Unless it's a whole fruit put into a juicer with the pulp, the fibre will be taken out, as well as the full nutritional value of that fruit, that you believe that you are consuming and what will be left is just sugar.

The issue that I have with drinking smoothies is: your body does not have to work as hard to digest the new calories taken in as there is a lack of fibre to slow the digestion process. In terms of boosting glucose, this is the opposite of what we want to do for weight loss.

Most people only put what tastes nice, into their smoothies, not what is good for their bodies nutritionally.

You may as well eat small amounts of all the things that you will put into the smoothie, and get the fibre to burn the calories while eating. Whenever you can do so, eat your food, don't drink it!

Protein shakes are not the best option. A protein shake will contain additives, preservatives, flavourings, sugars, and yes loads of protein, leaving out other nutritional elements that you will need to get from eating actual food proteins.

Flavoured water is NOT water. It is not a step up to water or a tasty alternative to water. If you squeeze a strawberry, blackberry raspberry or lemon the juice never comes out clear. Don't try to fool yourself by drinking a chemically modified drink and saying that it is water. It simply is not.

DON'T GET SAUCY!

So you think you've got your eating down to an art, and you've accounted for your low calorie meal. For example: your steak is 150 calories, potatoes are 90 calories and your greens & vegetables are 50 calories. You've made it!.. The perfect calorie intake. So what do you do? You go and add a tablespoon of some peppercorn sauce, at 6.2

grams, to go with your steak (112 calories) and of course you have to have some mayonnaise - why not, it's only 10 grams (42 calories) - and a couple glasses of white wine. 502 calories extra won't hurt. So now you've added to your meal of 290 calories, an additional 656 calories making your meal 946 calories.

Now I'm not saying don't eat sauce, but If you really think about it, your food shouldn't need sauce. If it's seasoned right. At the end of the day all you're doing when you add sauce to your food is adding sugar, and more than likely MSG. Now I ask, is that really worth it...

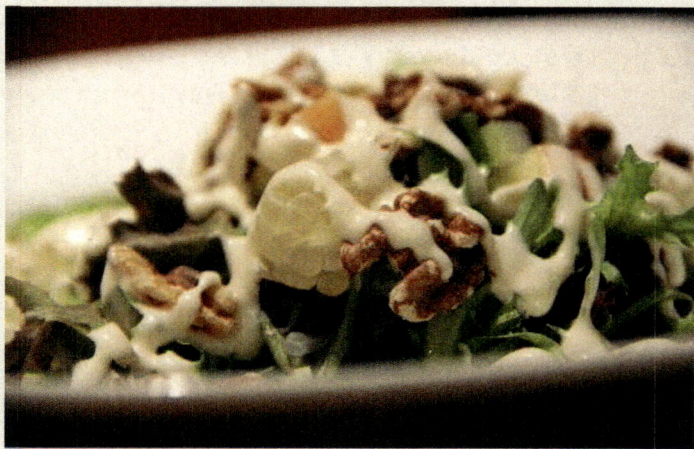

UNDERSTANDING SUGAR

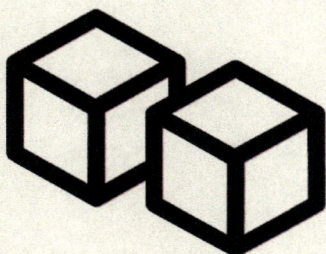

NO ADDED SUGAR

With our daily allowance being 20 grams maximum, it is easy to see why so many of us find it hard to cut sugar out of our diets. How do we wean ourselves from this highly addictive preserve? Sugar has no nutritional value, it is 100% carbohydrate, 5 times as addictive as cocaine, and in absolutely everything we eat, so we cannot avoid it, nor completely wean ourselves off of it.

However, what we can do is use it in an appropriate way. Let's look at the pros and cons of sugar. Ask yourself the following questions, before consuming what you are about to eat or drink.

Does It taste good? Are you actually tasting the food, or drink that you're consuming... or are you consuming the MSG flavour, or the sugar put into the product. If you had the ingredients to make what you are about to eat in front of you, would it taste just as good?

The truth is, without the added sodium and excess sugar in the sweet snacks we drink or eat, we probably wouldn't eat them if we had to make them ourselves.

Just like MSG, sugar will stimulate your dopamine receptors, where-as MSG is just sodium, so it does not have as much of an addictive effect on your brain. Which in excess can raise your blood pressure.

However sugar will transform into excess glucose in the body, which will convert to fat, spike insulin levels, causing dehydration in the brain and body. The results of which puts a strain on your liver, pancreas, thyroid, (your body's thermostat that regulates your body temperature) which in turn causes you to burn fat quickly or much slower.

Why not just eat watermelon, berries and strawberries, blueberries, even an apple or orange now and again when you crave something sweet. All these fruits carry fibre and nutrition that your body will break down, to use much better, and add more nutritional value, than just sugar alone, which will make extra glucose that will turn into fat in your body.

If sugar cannot be used immediately / appropriately at the point in time required, The feeling that can **sugar** give you will create a spike in energy. This is always short lived, as simple sugars convert to glucose so fast, and you'll get a rush from the glucose stimulating the brain's dopamine receptors. Also the sugar crashes, as your brain can only process a certain amount. This can take place, within a 20 minute period.

Glucose mixed with liquid, will be absorbed 10 times faster, as there is nothing to slow down the digestion process. It is much better if you get sustained energy from eating foods rich in good fats, such as avocados, coconut oil (with MCT that is good for brain function), olives, and dark chocolate (rich in magnesium). All these good fats will lower cholesterol levels, give longer sustained vibrancy, without a spike then dip in energy as they don't go through the pancreas .

It is important to remember, whatever stimulants that we put into our bodies, our brains will be affected. Your brain will automatically try to find a way to balance the excess chemicals . In this case, the excess sugar is the over-stimulant. The brain will try to get rid of or convert the unneeded sugar as quickly as possible, and take however long that it needs to process, so that it can restore balance in the body. The by-product of this is glucose being stored as fat for when it is needed.

If we take a look at a 1 litre bottle of coke which contains 108g of sugar. That is over 5 times your body's required amount. You can start to see why there are people who can develop diabetes, bad skin conditions, and headaches so quickly. This can come from as little as 2 litre bottles of coke per day.

Well what about coke zero or diet coke or 0 calorie drinks? There are only 3 real 0 calorie drinks: water, tea, and coffee. The issue with these shop bought, 0-calorie fizzy drinks is a chemical called aspartame, this chemical is said to be 5 times as sweet as sugar, but also does not break down in the body the same way. It doesn't convert to glucose either. The question then is, what does aspartame do? The answer is nobody properly knows. A lot of studies point to aspartame being carcinogenic (cancerous) but the jury is still out on this one. If we take a look back in time, 30+ years ago, there was another chemical that we were told wasn't bad for us, known as nicotine, in cigarettes and cigars. I remember Super King adverts in the 90s, Hamlet cigars being promoted on TV. The jury was out then, of the effects of nicotine, on the brain and body. Well fast forward to the 2020s, now and the millions of people who died from nicotine poison, throat cancer,

C.O.P.D. and lung disease are insurmountable. Nowadays if you light a cigarette in public, you'd be looked on as a pariah. Well, it's a good job we still got vapes then... Lol, the jury's out on them too.artificial sugars If you can't go without sugar, there are always replacements. Inulin powder and stevia,which you can you to make cakes put in your tea, coffee or add to a homemade sorbet .

OWN YOUR GENETICS

I've competed in natural bodybuilding a total of 6 times and been placed high enough in all my shows to go through to a British final. I am 6 '2 and 92 kilos on stage, and while this may sound impressive to the average person, it is not the ideal metrics for a bodybuilder. 90% of the best natural bodybuilders stand at 5' 7 and will weigh between 90 and 95 kilos on stage.

Me going on stage against someone of the same weight

but 7 inches shorter, will make me look gangly and long limbed. I would need to be at least 105 kilos on stage to look impressive. This would require me to carry around more excessive weight. I would also have to force feed myself to gain the right amount of muscle, eating up to 6 or 7 meals a day.

In addition, I should be training to a standard that I am just not mentally prepared for, nor have the time or money to commit, It would take a toll on my body, trying to walk around off season at least 115 kilos, which I have never done in my life. I am already the biggest in my family, at 107 kilos, At some point I have to accept to do what was required to become a natural bodybuilder. I just didn't have the Genetics (naturally) or I was not willing to push my body beyond the limits that it took (Naturally). You can't be built like Arnold Schwarzenegger, Beyonce Knowles, Jennifer Lopez, or Anthony Joshua. Not unless you're related to them. So stop trying.

You can only be the best version of yourself. If you're 5,3 weighing 60kg, chances are you'll not become a basketball player, but you still could become a gymnast, a sprinter, or maybe a flyweight boxer.

You see the thing is, if you tend to chase what you like the look of, rather than your potential, or your physical attributes, you can end up missing the bigger picture.

As a female, you may be more suited to a curvy fuller physique, let's say, you are a size 16, chasing a dress size 6, because you've been influenced by social media, friends or a significant other. You may feel good in the

47

short term. While it is possible to achieve this look. It could potentially make you feel uncomfortable, lethargic and become more hassle in the long term healthwise. This could Lead to new complications that you may not have gambled on, such as body dysmorphia, Anorexia or Bulimia. I've worked with clients' who have the ability to put on muscle very quickly. Even while being naturally curvy at a size 8 or 16, they still want to be super thin. Despite their frame being completely different to what they want to look like, as their genetic background simply doesn't consist of a slim body composition within their family tree. Try as they may, a size 6 is not on the cards for them. In my opinion, why try to look like a copy of someone else, when you can make your uniqueness stand out 10 times better. You are the only one in the world that looks like you, so own it.

Whether you were a size 6, 10, 28, or 32 waistline when you were 18 or 21 in the growing stages of your life. You're not now. Although you may be able to get down to those inches, chances are your body composition will more than likely have changed. So a size 10 person, whose body has grown wider, and stretched skin, put on excess muscle and fat, with middle-aged spread, may not look as good physically, as it sounds when they finally achieve that goal and are standing in the mirror. Learn to love the skin you're in. You never know you could look a lot better with thicker thighs and a fuller bum. The thing is, no matter what you look like on the outside confidence comes from within so learn to love yourself.

You're only going to be stuck with this body for the rest of your life. So if you don't like it now, you can't buy a new one. You can only make this one look better and the chances are the bits you don't like about yourself nobody actually will think twice about. Women 16 to 26: Being a lady at this stage in your life is extremely hard. Like the boys, becoming aware of your sexuality, you may feel societal pressure. You may feel the urge to conform to the beauty standards of the current time depending on your friendship group, culture, race and sexual preference.

You may become torn between the body you want, and the body that fits your lifestyle and social setting. Your training may also be affected by similar pressures. Your thought processing will be affected by social status, as well as social media way more, due to hormones and the fact that your brain has not yet fully matured.

So my main advice here would be the same as for the young male's in your age range. Look at training and exercise as an outlet primarily for your health. Do the exercises that make you feel good. Sports, training and dieting go hand in hand with one another. For a developing brain, having a sport or exercise routine will work wonders. Focus, discipline, structure and most importantly direction is what is needed in any young person's life.

In my view, any type of exercise - let it be boxing, football, dancing, athletics or even martial arts - provides a good solution to helping insecurity, lack of confidence, low self esteem.

Take your advice from a close responsible person who cares, over any kind of social media or your peers.When it comes to exercise in the gym, it is best to prioritise mobility flexibility first and strength secondary. swimming , circuit training, and low resistance training is the best approach, when it comes to training.

The disadvantage most women will face during their training life is the cycle of your period and ovulation. During your period you may become lethargic, emotional, and feel weak. In opposition during ovulation you will feel strong, energetic , happy you will be less likely to have stomach bloating and at some point feel like you are at your physical peak.

Women 26 to 40: It's all about lifting heavy, while paying attention to where you are in your cycle. In the lead up to ovulation (**luteal phase**) you want to be doing more heavy lifting, going for PBs. Whereby after ovulation (follicular phase), approaching your period, it would be best to increase your cardio. You could go for 1 hour as a standard, 3 times per week, instead of your regular 40 minutes.

When it comes to training, the recommended frequency is 3 times per week for new starters. More advanced trainers can go for 4 to 5 times per week and elite trainers would practise 5 times per week, twice a day.

It is necessary to consider the increased risks of training, at time of pregnancy and the period shortly after giving birth.

During these times, hernia is 3 times more likely in women, due to the linea alba (the band of tissue that sits underneath and between the abdominals) becoming very weak.

There are breathing exercises you can do to strengthen the deeper abdominal wall. During pregnancy, it is best to avoid traditional sit ups and any exercises such as crunches or mountain climbers. Best to opt for controlled breathing techniques, bird dogs, or standing core exercises. Other than that, most movements during pregnancy are a good idea.

There will be caveats and outliers in all categories as we are all individuals. I've trained women in their 60s and 70s stronger and fitter than most men in their 30s. On the other hand, there are women who had early menopause, as young as 30. Not for one second do I say that a woman can be judged on her age alone to determine how she should and must train.

When it comes to health and fitness, people in general can never be generalised. Where biology is concerned, women tend to be more-so affected by losing bone density, osteoarthritis, after menopause, which usually can start around the age of 40. During pregnancy women can develop gestational diabetes which may put them at risk of diabetes after pregnancy. If a woman gets pregnant after the age of 36, this is considered as geriatric pregnancy. It is common for women past this age to have smaller babies due to less nutrients being fed to the baby. **women 40+**to 60 When you are entering menopause, lift heavy and stick with your compound lifts, Squats, Deadlift, Clean and Press barbell. As a woman approaching menopause, you'll need to build bone density as your bones tend to become brittle during this time in your life.

Lifting heavy will help increase much needed muscle mass and improve your body composition. Training 3 times per week for up to an hour per time will be the best thing I can recommend. When it comes to cardiovascular exercise, I would suggest the stairmaster or a treadmill on incline or a bike on high resistance. 40 minutes minimum to an hour also works 3 to 4 times per week, but this is still not a one size fits all solution. When it comes to women 40+ as your hormones will wreak havoc with your moods and cortisol levels; Not to mention if you have underlying conditions such as P.C.O.S. Endometriosis training may be the last thing on your mind.

The tail end of periods, luteal phase or follicular phase beginning. You ladies have a lot to contend with. It's bad enough knowing that you're born with all the eggs you produce in your body are about to run out. Now you have to deal with hot flushes and feeling irritating discomfort, for what seems like no reason. Training relatively heavy will help to build bone density, improve much needed muscle and strength. Also ease some of the complexities of menopause, lower stress levels.

Men 16 to 26: You're still growing, your brain doesn't stop forming until you're 26 years old, your body doesn't stop growing until 21. Your testosterone levels are through the roof and if not then speak with your doctor. But very similar to men 26 to 36 you can do what you like, but I would recommend taking your time to learn your craft, enjoy training, learn what types of training styles is best for you.

Avoid taking advice from Tik Tok. If you're ever offered steroids then remember steroids are synthetic testosterone once you add this to your body, your natural testosterone production shuts down as your body doesn't want to over produce, so only use steroids, if you have consulted with your doctor, even if you feel that you may be underdeveloped. You still have time. Everyone grows at different rates.

I remember being at school and having boys in my class with full beards and chest hair at the age of 14. I remember boys with six packs and mountains of muscle at 15, but fast forward 10, 15, 20 years later those same people seem to have aged in dog years. Some of those guys were bald by 19 and had beer bellies by 21. My point is people can peak at different rates.

Hormones and puberty can have the same sort effect on girls as well. Some girls peaked at 18 and didn't change much, whereas the late bloomers ended up looking amazing at 40 plus.

I'd like to think I sit somewhere in the middle. Social media is not the best place to get advice from a jacked role model. Treat social media like entertainment and not a place to get wisdom. Research and research some more. Speak with people who will deter you from rushing into things. Rather than a person who will sensationalise.

Men 26 to 40: Literally the prime of your life, this is the time you pack on as much muscle as possible, you can lift as heavy as possible and train how you want. You are the silverback Kings of the gym, at this stage, enjoy it. Treat your body well, eat plenty of vegetables and protein, and drink lots of water.

If you're new to lifting, or have been doing this for some time. The best lifts you should be doing are the deadlift.

If you're a man (XY), you may benefit from losing excess fat around your lower tummy region, as excess belly fat will lower your testosterone levels, so this should be paramount for you to get as low as possible, not for aesthetics, but for your health.

It is important that you make your core as strong as possible to prevent umbilical hernias which is common amongst men. So a strong core is a must. It will also help you to avoid lower back pain. You don't need to have a six pack but you do need a strong core.

Besides a strong core for anyone, learning how to train can be a bit of a conundrum, so I've listed some key points below in the table that you can follow:

Men 40 - 60: 45 minute, high intensity workouts are the best thing for fat loss.

Short breaks in between sets, moderate weights and a full body training at least 2 times per week with a touch up of your favourite body parts once a week. You can still do cardio up to 40 minutes on the back of your workout or 3 more times per week, but training longer where cardiovascular exercise is concerned, will eat into your muscle mass instead of reducing fat. Training longer than

45 minutes if you're a man (XY chromosome) in the 40+ range, can increase Cortisol levels in the body and have the opposite effect of what you want to achieve. Let the young boys have the gym and the heavy weights.

While it is impossible to cover the fitness needs of every group and individual in a single book, there is a specific type of people I want to highlight, regardless of their age group., Those who are considered obese or morbidly obese. Your journey will undertake a lot more complexity from anxiety, stress, lethargy, and mental anguish. I suggest counselling alongside your fitness training. You will need to understand that your goal will not only be about losing weight. It will also be about maintaining the weight that you have lost and how to deal with a lot of loose skin you may have gained as a result. What do you do now with this new body you have? Setting up a plan of action, and acting like your life depends on you not failing, is the best approach to have in my eyes.

Measure your progress weekly and treat every small win as a win regardless. Go out and buy yourself a new item of clothing once you've met your size goal marker. For example: you've dropped a dress size, buy a new dress; you've lost inches on your waist, buy a smaller pair of jeans. Throw away your old clothing, take pictures weekly. Make plans as though you have lost the weight already. Save money for your surgery once you have lost the weight, as you may have to deal with a lot of loose skin. Give yourself extra time and only compete with the person you were yesterday, because that is the only person that truly matters.

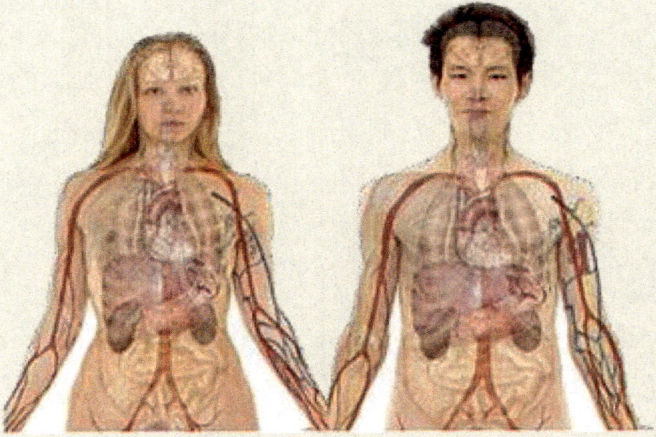

The table below is a guide, pertaining to training within a gym setting, using resistance training as part of your main workout routine. Circuit training can also be used in combination with resistance training as well as high intensity training. This table refers to individuals, who fall into a bodyfat percentage between 15% and up to 30%. If you do fall out of this range, you still will be able to use advice from the table, however times may need to be reviewed, to accommodate to bodyfat percentages.

	Women 16-26	Women 26-40	Women 40-60	Men 16-26	Men 26-40	Men 40-60
No# of days training per week Time per day	5-7 times 1.5 hours	3-5 times 1.5-2 hours	3 times 1.5 hours	5-7 times 1.5-2 hours	3-7 times 1.5-2 hours	3-5 times 40 mins- 1 hour
Best exercise recommended	Light weight /full body	Any type of training you wish	Compound lifting strength training	Any type of training you wish	Compound lifting strength training Deadlifts, and the seated row single arm without a chest support	Light weight /full body circuit training
Challenges you may face	Your body is still developing so don't do any exercises that involves heavy lifting	You are susceptible to periods and ovulation so it is best to structure your rest periods, cardio and diet around these times, pregnancy core training will need to adjust	Menopause Bone density and muscle density may be low so don't be tempted to lift beyond your R.P.E. of 60% 8-12 rep range	While your body is developing your tendons can be at risk of tears if muscles develop too quickly	A boost in testosterone could cause you to want to over train your body and cause long term injury	Training for more than 1 hour at a time may increase cortisol and increase fatigue

Benefits	You give yourself time to develop mobility and strength at the same try and develop muscle memory	Low resistance training can encourage muscle growth it is recommended that sports and mobility training can help develop a balanced physique	Training this way could help boost testosterone levels strengthen bones build muscle reduce fat storage	Testosterone will help you to develop muscle quick	If you stick to a planned programme which includes a deload week you will be able to optimise strength gains and longevity	Retain muscle, burn fat, increase mobility Unless you are completely new to resistance training you will continue to see massive gains with consistency
Type of training recommended	Football Athletics Dance Swimming	Weight lifting Crossfit Hiit Swimming Athletics Swimming	Weightlifting Aerobics Yoga Pilates Natural Bodybuilding Swimming	Athletics Weightlifting Crossfit Powerlifting Natural Bodybuilding Swimming	Athletics Weightlifting Crossfit Powerlifting Natural Bodybuilding Football Swimming	Natural Bodybuilding Hiit Swimming Yoga Resistance training
Priority	Flexibility Mobility	Mobility Diet Build muscle	Diet Build muscle Mobility	Flexibility Mobility Build muscle	Diet Mobility Build muscle	Maintain Muscle Mobility
Goal overall	Increase mobility	Build muscle Maintain flexibility	Build bone density	Increase mobility	Build muscle	Maintain adequate testosterone levels

One Man's Meat, Another Man's Poison

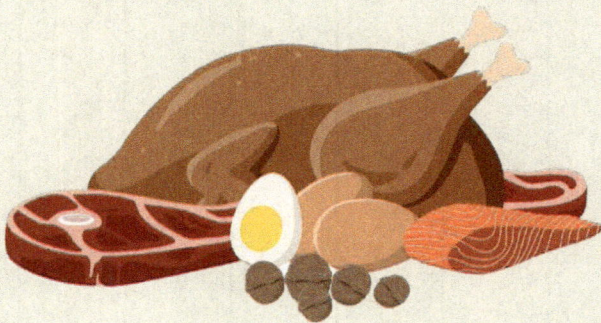

So you've been training for a while now, you're absolutely killing it at the gym. You are eating healthy, doing your cardio 5 times a week. Ticking all your boxes.

However there still seems to be one or two things wrong. You notice that after your nine Eggs for breakfast you become bloated, or whenever you've eaten your lovely red bell peppers for breakfast - like your amazing Personal Trainer, Phil has recommended - you get severe stomach cramps or diarrhoea.

This is strange as you've never gotten these symptoms before. This would have been a major issue in the past, but you have made up your mind that you're going to stick with your new diet plan, despite what your body is telling you. Plus PT Phil knows absolutely everything about food. Surely he can't be wrong about diet? I mean look at him... He eats nine eggs and red bell peppers a day and he looks amazing...

Well here's the thing, Phil may not be allergic to

capsaicin (the active component in peppers). Phil may also not have mentioned how he chooses to cook his eggs, by boiling them, instead of frying them now, like he used to. All because he developed an allergy to olives and can no longer cook his food in olive oil. When things like this happen, it may be time to go back to the drawing board.

There are several different approaches we can use. The first is a food allergy test, you can buy some really good kits online. The second option is not something that I'd personally do as an option. I've heard from other coaches and read some old studies that are a bit more extreme and controversial, that you can use your to determine **blood type** how your diet should work. This option can produce a moral dilemma. If for example, you are a practising vegan, but according to your blood type reading, you should be eating meat in your diet. There are also tests you can do to find this out as well, but as I mentioned the research is old and can be considered controversial

The third thing you can do is, the process of elimination in your diet. Start by taking away particular ingredients that you may use in your meal prep, then track your results week by week. You may well find that you have developed an intolerance to a particular food or you could have already been allergic from the beginning. Some fun facts:

- 2.3% of adults in the U.K. are allergic to cow's milk or lactose intolerant. **allergy stats**,

- 0.5% of adults in the U.K. are allergic to eggs,

0.3% of adults are allergic to soy, chickpeas and nuts/ legumes.

- 3% of adults and up to as much as 10.3% of adults in the U.K. (depending on the diagnosis) will be allergic to shellfish. 0.5% of adults in the

U.K. have a wheat and gluten intolerance

KING OF THE LIFTS

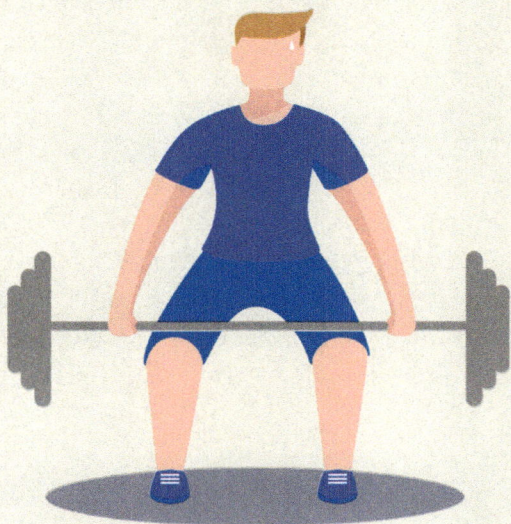

If there was only one exercise that you could do in the gym, it would be the **Deadlift**, whether you are training for sports, bodybuilding, losing fat, gaining muscle, boosting testosterone, improving your posture. The risk - reward ratio is minimal, and with proper form - not training with ego - if you can't lift the weight properly, the most that will happen, is that you just can't lift it. And if you manage to lift it you can just drop it if you come unstuck.

The deadlift remains the king in my opinion. No other compound movement will hit as many muscles in the body as this exercise. If you are new to training make this a staple part of your routine, and I don't limit this advice to just young people. Honestly it works well for young, old people, also people who are new to training at any age or level, and any gender.

This is the best lift you can do and once perfected will give you the most bang for your buck. The deadlift will stimulate your entire posterior chain/ all the muscles throughout the back of your body and the muscles that are responsible for keeping your posture straight.

That being said, there is one other exercise which is better, the only issue with this, is that it has a higher risk factor, which is why I can't put it as number 1. The Clean and Press will use the same muscles as the Deadlift and also include the shoulders, triceps, Biceps and upper chest.

You can't go as heavy as the deadlift, but honestly you don't need to. Between 5 to 8 working repetitions at 60% of rate of perceived exertion (R.P.E) for 4 sets, and resting for 90 to 120 seconds between sets, will be enough to feel the benefits. You can actually use this same approach with the Deadlift as well.

My third best exercise and quite honestly the exercise I love to hate, because mentally this is the most challenging, and very high risk compound of all the exercises is the barbell squat.

The Barbell squat requires technique, form, core strength control, as well as a mindset and focus for every rep. For safety you need a spotter. when attempting near to your RPE. In fact if you're in the range of 50% it's time to look for a spotter with the squat, simply because there are so many factors that can go wrong. If you're a beginner, use a squat rack with safety bars to minimise risk. And aim for your rest to be 120+ seconds, because this exercise requires full concentration.

If you're new to lifting, this will be one of the most challenging exercises you can do and for this reason you will see a ton of people avoiding this movement. You can usually spot them a mile away, the people with big upper bodies. Slim legs and lots of excuses as to why they don't squat.

When it comes to circuit training I would use much lighter weights and my RPE would come down to 20%, as the goal would be to do as many reps as I can within a specific timing and with consideration of my rest period (of 15 to 20 seconds).

While doing a circuit will be only long enough to replenish my ATP (Adenosine triphosphate) stores, enabling me enough time to recover and increase my endurance and stamina overall, then my need to go heavy and build strength is not my goal anymore. My goal is now to burn fat, use my fast twitch response, keep my heart rate up and my cardiovascular system at peak levels.

LET'S TALK SUPPLEMENTS...

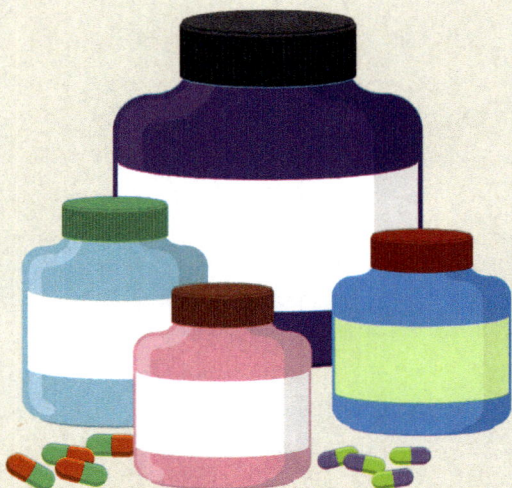

Creatine is my favourite muscle building performance enhancing supplement of all time. Taken with water, unflavoured powdered supplement, is the King's choice. 1 teaspoon of creatine would be the same as eating 5, 10 ounce steaks. Beta alanine is an amino acid and delays ATP and allows you to get extra reps, it will make you feel itchy as a side effect, but after a few weeks side effects will subside. Tribulus Terrestris and zinc, is third in line for men and it will boost your testosterone naturally by 0.37% but in combination with Horny Goat weed you will notice a difference in training as well as libido Magnesium can be found in 80%+ dark chocolate.

Magnesium Citrate will boost energy levels and help with

lethargy. In fact Magnesium Glycinate will help improve blood flow. It is very good for those pins and needles. Iron also helps improve energy levels, but I'd rather eat foods rich in iron than take the supplements, and we can also get iron from spinach, Vitamin D what can I say besides take it? We all need vitamin D as we don't get enough sun, good for hair and nails, energy levels, mood. Vitamin D will be in all dark green leafy vegetables, the list goes on... 5-htp: This is also an amino acid and helps with sleep, melatonin, mood and depression. As with all supplements the key is to not let your body get used to it so 3 months taking consistently then one month clear And as you see with the exception of the amino acids you can get all the advantages from the foods we eat anyway.

Remember everything we put into our bodies will have a side effect. Too much protein will give you protein wind, bad breath and constipation. Too much water drank too fast without planned breaks, will wash out minerals needed in your body and cause dizzy spells. Too much vitamin D can result a buildup of calcium in the body which can result in weakened bones and damaged kidneys

Absolutely everything will carry a side effect. The issue is not the use of the food but the overuse that will cause issues.

LET'S TALK ABOUT MY CHALLENGE

Let's talk about my challenge. I did a challenge for myself, to see if I could get as lean as possible, within as quick a time as possible. The result was a success. During my challenge the most shocking changes apart from the obvious physical ones, were the mental improvements I experienced, and the speed of the transformation. The reason for this quick, miraculous change was simply cutting out processed sugars, as well as sweets, drinks and cakes. Now let me just say, I wasn't someone who would gorge on sweets and chocolate, nor did I drink fizzy drinks by the gallon. I'd have a Lattè once or twice a week. Looking back this sounds like a lot, but because I was highly active, a small part of me figured that I can get away with eating like this.

I was prone to eating a Wispa bar, a cupcake or a yum yum, maybe drinking a latte now and then, or one or two Lucozade once a day.

To most people this seems like an average kind of week of bad eating, but I swear as soon as I stopped having all the above goodies, after the initial first 3 days of withdrawal from my sugary treats, my mood improved. My energy levels also improved. My fitness and recovery time improved after exercise. It became easy for me to quit my bad eating habits, because I kept a time-bound goal in mind. I aimed to form new eating habits to replace the old ones, changing milk chocolate for 85% dark chocolate, eating lots of berries and watermelon to quench the sugar cravings.

Even though I still ate takeaways, I chose the beneficial foods high in protein, or I had meals as close to whole food as possible. For example, I ate chicken shish kebab if I had not prepared food at home, or had seafood soup from the local Chinese takeaway. I ate lunch at the local pub and got a steak, jacket potato with peas and lettuce, and tomatoes.

Eating in this way excited me more, as I'd go out looking for alternatives that were helpful to my new eating regime. Eating breakfast only after I had completed my cardio also came with new added benefits, it was as though training in ketosis brought a new level of energy. It is hard to explain unless you've tried it. It can be linked to what's known as the runners high, only with the fact that I'd be feeling this amazing burst of energy and I did not consume anything other than a pint of water in the morning.

When it came to problem solving, my brain seemed to think more clearly and respond more rapidly than usual. This could have been from all the extra sardines that I had been eating, sardines being rich in omega 3 & 6 (vitamins that are very good for brain health). Or it could even have been the combination of swapping my regular vegetable oil for coconut oil and extra virgin olive oil.

Waking up in the morning, now came without aches or pains from training. My weight went from 107 kg to 99 kg within 7 days. This was also down to the fact I was doing two 40 minute cardio sessions a day as well as resistance training 5 days a week, for 1 hour per day, which meant that the rapid changes were evident.

The funny thing with my challenge was the feedback that I was getting. I'd get told "oh, you look younger, "oh you look older" or "oh, you look better with the weight off, or nah I don't like seeing you with the weight off now. Some people asked "Have you gotten bigger?" Some said I looked skinny. With all the different opposed opinions, the thing that helped me to focus, was even though people had something to say, I knew what they really were noticing, was a change. This helped me to understand that what I was doing, had been working. It also puts things in perspective about how people view me from the outside. The opinions of others are just that, only their opinions.

You see, if you follow other people's judgement, and perception of how you should be, you will never make yourself happy. Understand, you'll never make everyone who has an opinion on you happy. It is always best to focus on your own goals. Remember, if people start noticing change for good, or bad, at least they're noticing change. Whether they think the change is a good or bad thing, well that's just their personal opinion. your journey is your own. Enjoy your body. Treat it well, because until we can buy body parts from a store of some sort, you're stuck with it.

Learn how to love yourself first. By embracing the fact that we all have strength, as well as weakness, our insecurities shouldn't be able to hold us back from our goals, only if we allow them too. In most cases identifying your insecurities can become a benefit. Knowing when to ask for help will only help you learn something new. Admitting to yourself that you may need help can help you develop as a person, and trying to mask your issues will only allow them to grow with time, even eating away at you like a cancerous parasite.

If we can recognise that we are the only ones that can see our insecurities, then we can say "I'm the only one who

knows

that you're there! Nobody else can see you, so therefore I own you, bitch!"

Take what you have learned here and apply it to your life.

Now go ahead, set yourself your own challenge, put a time and date to all your goals, as well as a purpose, because all we have in this world, is our state of health, and our time left on this earth.

https://youtu.be/tHu1ju6ADHk

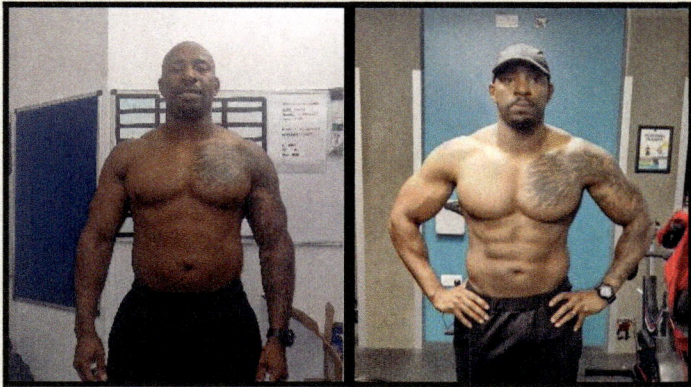

Pictures were taken 21 days apart

Thank you for reading, Philippe

Reference Page

Tips to cut Ghrelin:

ghrelin

Inflammation in the body:

Infhttps://www.webmd.com/diet/ss/slideshow-omega-3-health-benefits The secret seasoning: M.S.G.:

Understanding sugar:

https://pubmed.ncbi.nlm.nih.gov/23719144/https artificial sugars

https://www.nhs.uk/live-well/eat-well/food-types/how-does-sugar-in-our-diet-affect-our-health/#:~:text=Adults%20should%20have%20no%20more, day%2

Let's talk about supplements:

https://ods.od.nih.gov/factsheets/Magnesium-HealthProfessional/#:~:text=Magnesium%20is%20a%20cofactor%20in,

%2C%20 oxidative%20 phosphorylation%2C%20and%20 glycolysis. Own your genetics:

The phase of the menstrual cycle in women Luteal and follicular:(Females)

https://www.bupa.co.uk/newsroom/ourviews/strength-training-menopause

The secret seasoning:

Lemon juice Clearing your food from bacteria

ref:https://iopscience.iop.org/article/10.1088/1755-1315/217/1/012023

https://davidsuzuki.org/living-green/does-vinegar-kill-germs/#:~:text=Studies%20confirming%20vinegar's%20antibacterial%20properties,bactericidal%20activity%20increased%2 0with%20heat!

Inflammation in the body:

Cereals cereals

One man's meat: food allergies

https://health.clevelandclinic.org/blood-type-diet   Food allergy:

allergy stats

Lets talk supplements

://www.ncbi.nlm.nih.gov/pmc/articles/PMC4120469/#

:~:text=The%20results%20did%2 0not%20shohttpsw,free%20testosterone%20following

%20ingestion%20of

Printed in Great Britain
by Amazon

49282316R00046